THE HEART TEST THAT COULD SAVE YOUR LIFE

LM CLAY

The Heart Test That Could Save Your Life by L M Clay

(c) L M Clay 2019

All rights reserved. No portion of this book may be reproduced in any form without permission from the publisher, except as permitted by U.S. copyright law.

About the Author

About the author

The author is not a doctor but simply a person who watched so many family and friends struggle and sometimes die from heart disease. He simply decided to research and see if he could find a test that could be preventative in nature. To his surprise there was one that he didn't know about and is not as well known as many others.

This book is intended to educate those who don't know about this test and could benefit from it and quite possibly save their life.

Contents

Medical Disclaimer	7
Introduction	9
What This Book is About	13
1. What is Heart Disease	15
2. What is a Heart Attack?	17
3. Why Do Arteries Become Blocked?	21
4. Does Everyone Get Heart Disease?	25
5. Do You Need Treatment for Heart Disease?	29
6. Which Test Should You Have?	35
7. What is a Calcium Scoring Test	37
8. Who Uses the Calcium Score?	41
9. Why Don't We Take Steps to Help Ourselves?	45
10. Why Do We Ignore Medical Advice	47
11. What are the Treatments for Heart Disease?	53
12. Which Diet Should You Follow?	55
13. Different Approaches to Diet	57
14. Specific Food Types	63
15. Drug Treatment	69
16. One Hundred and Fifty Minutes of Fun	73
Afterword	75
Medical Terms You Should Understand	77
Notes	79

Medical Disclaimer

This information is not intended as medical advice or for prevention, diagnosis and treatment of medical issues, and should not be used as a substitute for professional medical advice, diagnosis, or treatment. Please consult your health care professional before considering any new dietary, diagnostics, or treatment options.

While we attempt to keep our information accurate and up to date, we cannot guarantee it is an accurate representation of the latest information regarding heart disease. I am not a medical practitioner and the opinions herein are my own.

Introduction

According to the Centers for Disease Control and Prevention (CDC) heart disease is the number one cause of death in the USA today for both men and women.[1] Over 600,000 people die from heart disease every year, that's one person, every minute of every hour of every day, every day of the year. And that is despite enormous leaps in medical science over the last 30-50 years.

For many the result is a painful, frightening heart attack which changes their life.

For some it's even more devastating.

A hale and healthy family member, someone's much loved father, mother, brother or sister, goes out one day and never comes back. It seems to come from nowhere, they had no symptoms, no reason to think they were at all unwell. The shock

Introduction

of an untimely, unexpected death can devastate a family and the worst thing about it is that most of us know a family where this has happened.

Recently a friend of mine who is only 39 was playing pick up hockey when he starting feeling weak and decided to lay down in the locker room. Luckily one of his friends called for an ambulance and that ended up saving my friend's life. His heart literally stopped twice in the ambulance and once in the hospital. He did survive and is doing fine today but had no previous signs of heart disease.

Another person I know was struggling to breathe and was taken to the hospital in a car. Unfortunately he died on the way. He was only 48 years old. The Doctor at the emergency room told his relatives the heart attack was so massive he would have died even if he had reached the hospital in time.

My mother died of a heart attack in the hospital while being treated for diabetes, my father died from a heart attack while being treated for cancer. My brother has had two angioplasty operations on clogged arteries or he too would most likely have passed away at just 58.

Death is only one possible outcome from heart disease. Heart disease can leave you unfit and unable to cope with your job or your normal life.

Introduction

It is especially terrifying because it seems to come from nowhere. But is heart disease truly an invisible killer? Are there really no warning signs?

Doctors are convinced they can tell those at risk from heart disease and at some point you are likely to encounter the many tests in use. Even though you have no symptoms of heart disease the tests may be administered as part of your annual physical or almost any medical examination.

From 2005 to 2015 the death rate from heart disease decreased. This may have been the result of extensive screening and early treatment when the disease was still asymptomatic, but in recent years progress has slowed. Given the number of new surgical techniques, new drugs hitting the market, the reduction in smoking and increase in air quality, this is surprising. Blood tests like cholesterol screening have become even more common in the last few years, more and more Americans take drugs for high blood pressure and to reduce cholesterol, but still the rate of heart disease stays high leading some practitioners to believe that the tests and subsequent treatment may not be as effective as originally believed.

We owe it to ourselves to remain educated on this subject in order to engage with health professionals in an informed discussion about the prevention and possible treatment of heart disease. Our doctors care deeply about our well being, no-one doubts that, but no one cares about you as much as *you* do.

    L M Clay (hearttest@yahoo.com)

What This Book is About

Almost every week one or other piece of research into cardiovascular disease is described in the media. In the week I started this book there were many articles on the link between diet drinks and heart disease, with one newspaper making a case for us all to abandon soft drinks altogether and take to water.

At the same time the soft drink industry maintains there is no problem. Who is right and how do you decide?

Ultimately your health is your business. You may take the view that since the information is so contradictory, all you can do is ignore it all, but would your family agree?

This book is designed to help you become better informed about cardiovascular disease, what it is, where it comes from, what the treatments are and whether you should be concerned.

It is not a replacement for medical advice, nor does it pretend to provide any.

What this book hopes to do is increase your awareness of the subject, encourage you to ask questions, seek answers, take an active part in your medical care before following any advice, whether it comes from the internet, your best friend, the newspapers or your doctor.

1

What is Heart Disease

Heart Disease is a general term which covers many conditions or illnesses. The most common form of heart disease is CVD or cardiovascular disease. Typically this is not a problem with the heart itself but with the blood vessels which surround it. The best way to understand what it is, is to take a look at the heart and how it works.

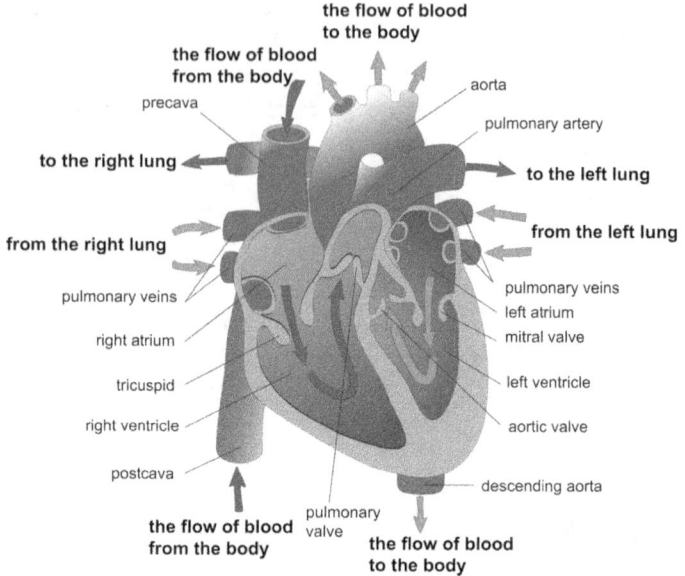

Your heart is a double pump where one side pushes blood around the body and the other half pushes blood through the lungs. It is essentially a large muscle with no chemical function, but don't be fooled. Your heart is vital, it's just that unlike other bodily organs (eyes, ears, kidneys for example) human beings only have one. We need to take care of it.

2

What is a Heart Attack?

Like any other muscle in your body, your heart can be badly damaged if it doesn't receive an adequate supply of blood. If the supply is suddenly cut off your heart can stop beating, blood containing oxygen won't reach your brain and you'll lose consciousness. The muscle tissue of your heart will be injured, weakening the heart-muscle as a whole.

This is what we call a heart attack and doctors call a myocardial infarction or MI.

The most common cause of heart attack is blockage in one of the coronary arteries. The most common cause of a blocked artery is a blood clot in an artery which has already been reduced in size as a result of atherosclerosis.[1]

Heart attacks can also be caused by slow blood

flow, as happens when your heart is beating very fast or you have low blood pressure. If your demand for oxygen is higher than the supply, a heart attack can be the result.

Any weakness in your heart will damage your whole cardiovascular system. As your body degrades with age, elderly people are more likely to suffer heart attacks.

Blood

The average person contains around 5 litres of blood, a stream of fluid which circulates through your heart carrying oxygen and nutrients to your cells and taking waste products away. In addition to oxygen and nutrients your blood contains white blood cells which fight infection and platelets which help your blood to clot when necessary.

When your body needs more oxygen your heart beats faster sending more oxygen per second to your muscles. If you encounter an infection the same thing happens. Your heart beats to deliver blood containing immune cells to fight off the invasion.

Without blood and the oxygen your red blood cells contain, the cells of your body will die. Your heart is no exception. The cells will be damaged every time your blood flow is inadequate or interrupted. A blockage is usually experienced as pain.

If the blood supply is cut off you are likely to lose consciousness.

When doctors discuss cardiovascular disease they make it sound as though its all about your heart. In reality it is more about your blood.[2]

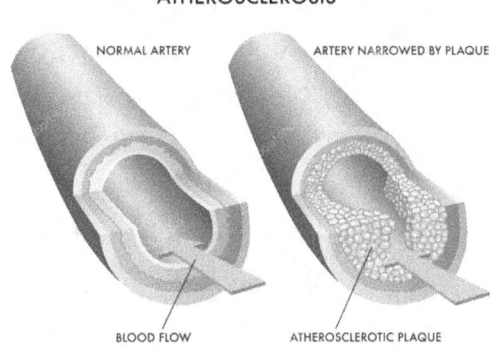

ATHEROSCLEROSIS

Blood has three major constituents:

- Red blood cells. Constantly produced in your bone marrow, red blood cells are the most common cell in the blood, but they are also highly unusual as they have no nucleus. This unusual configuration allows red blood cells to store more haemoglobin, the chemical which transports oxygen throughout the body.[3]
- Plasma Makes up 60% of your blood and is mainly water. Contains proteins

(albumin, clotting factors, antibodies, enzymes and hormones) Contains sugars (glucose) and fat particles.
- White Blood Cells and platelets are the body's shock troops. They circulate in the blood until they are needed due to some of damage to the body or the presence of an infection. Lymphocytes, Monocytes, Granulocytes, Neutrophils, Eosinophils, Basophils

Also circulating in your blood are fats or lipids including cholesterol. The level of cholesterol in your blood is something doctors use to tell whether you are developing heart disease and whether you need treatment.

3

Why Do Arteries Become Blocked?

This is another circumstance where the medical jargon can be especially confusing. *Arteriosclerosis* refers to the thickening of the walls of the arteries which usually occurs as we get older. *Atherosclerosis* is something quite different and can occur at any age when artery walls are damaged leading to the formation of plaque.

Plaque on the inside of your arteries is made from several substances which circulate in your blood. Cholesterol usually gets the blame, but is actually just one of many substances which can form plaque. These include calcium, fat, cholesterol, cellular waste and fibrin. Many internet sources name foods as the guilty party when it comes to blocked arteries and fatty foods or foods containing cholesterol are the big bogeyman. However, scientists now know that most blood cholesterol is produced by the liver. Rather than avoid foods high in cholesterol, doctors suggest avoiding foods high in saturated fat as many believe these foods are responsible for stimulating the liver to produce cholesterol.[1]

The question doctors can't answer is what starts the process of plaque deposits. It seems to be connected to damage in the lining of the artery wall, but there are many possible reasons for the damage to occur. Doctors believe high blood pressure, for example, increases the rate at which plaque builds up as does diabetes or smoking cigarettes.

The biggest problem with clogged arteries is that you won't experience any symptoms until something major happens, like a stroke or heart attack.

If the artery is more than 70% clogged you might suffer symptoms like chest pain (also known as angina), shortness of breath, heart palpitations, weakness, nausea or sweating. Since these symptoms can be associated with many very different conditions, doctors have developed many different tests to determine whether arteries are actually clogged, these vary from cholesterol screening to ultrasounds scans, and MRI or PET scan CT scan or cardiac stress test.

If you do have clogged arteries there are many possible forms of treatment depending on the severity of the problem. These range from diet and lifestyle changes to surgeries of different kinds and medication.[2]

The problem is, you won't know your arteries are clogged until one day when it makes a difference. Why take drugs for a condition you may not have? This question often comes up when you have a family history of heart disease. In this case Doctors will consider you at risk for heart disease even if you have never experienced any symptoms. If you are also diabetic, obese or both, your doctor may go into overdrive suggesting a number of tests and/or treatments and you may take the view that it's better to be safe than sorry.

The simplest and safest thing to do is to **assume you do have a problem** and modify your lifestyle accordingly, but the truth is, you won't. The situation is not unlike being an addict. **You know what you need to do, you just can't bring yourself to do it.** The drive is coming from your doctor, not from you.

The only way to change that is to become

informed. Learn about the risk factors for heart disease and how they apply to you and your family. **Until the desire for change comes from you, not your doctor, the likelihood of real and lasting change is very low.**

4

Does Everyone Get Heart Disease?

Heart disease is not inevitable and there are measures we can all take to avoid it. The mortality rate from cardiovascular disease has improved enormously. The question is, why?

According to some,[1] this was due to the dietary guidelines for the USA published in 1977. A review of current eating habits indicates that these guidelines have had some success in changing American eating patterns with carbohydrate consumption increasing while fat consumption decreased over the same period.

The question to ask is whether this change is for the better. The reduction in premature death from heart disease seems to show the change has been for the better, but many things have changed over the same period and these may be more significant, for example smoking has decreased, lead has been removed from petrol, air quality has improved and so has medical treatment.

Sadly the improvement in mortality rates seems to have stalled in both the USA and the UK where deaths from heart disease actually increased in 2018. There have, at the same time, been major increases in obesity and diabetes in both countries, resulting in the following statement in the journal Nutrition:

> Since 1971, the shift in macronutrient share from fat to carbohydrate is primarily due to an increase in absolute consumption of carbohydrate as opposed to a change in total fat consumption. General adherence to recommendations to reduce fat consumption has coincided with a substantial increase in obesity.[2]

As a result some have suggested that the shift to a low-fat, carbohydrate rich diet may be *responsible* for this increase, that the dietary recommendations have not been beneficial and may even have increased the risks of cardiovascular disease.

This makes it even more important that you are aware not just of the dietary guidelines, but that you have the basic facts about this complex area of medicine. Only then can you, with your doctor's advice, make informed decisions about your health and your treatment.

5

Do You Need Treatment for Heart Disease?

Doctors across the USA and the rest of the world regularly test cholesterol levels in their patients and may, after seeing the results, suggest further treatment, either through behavioral changes, drugs or other medical procedures.

Here's Why.

Just over thirty years ago two American doctors, Michael S Brown and Jospeh L Goldstein won the Nobel prize for medicine, the prize was awarded for their work in understanding cholesterol. A new age had dawned with a new level of understanding for cardiovascular disease (CVD) and how high levels of cholesterol could accumulate and clog arteries leading to heart attacks and strokes. The world now had a new medical bogeyman.

Since then doctors have measured cholesterol levels in their patients in an attempt to predict who needs treatment for heart disease, but how reliable are cholesterol levels when it comes to predicting heart disease?

Cholesterol

Cholesterol is a perfectly normal constituent of blood and can be found in the membrane of every cell in your body.[1] There are two sources of cholesterol; your liver and the food you eat. Animal products, like meat, fish and eggs contain cholesterol, while plant based products do not. Cholesterol is a normal and essential part of the body where it helps to produce vitamin D, insulate nerve cells, produce bile, maintain cell membranes and produce hormones, so why do doctors seem so obsessed by it?

High Density Lipoprotein (HDL)

High density lipoprotein (HDL) combines with cholesterol and carries it back to the liver so it can be flushed out of your body. Because it carries cholesterol away, HDL is sometimes known as 'good' cholesterol.

Low Density Lipoprotein (LDL)

Various studies have shown that high levels of

LDL are related to the development of clogged arteries hence it has been called 'bad' cholesterol.

As doctors studied the role of cholesterol they found that high levels of HDL were not a problem, in fact they seem to protect the arteries by carrying the LDL away and stimulating repair of the endothelium or artery walls. Total cholesterol is not, hence a good measure of future risk of heart disease, however high levels of LDL combined with low levels of HDL, might be.

In a 2014 study[2] researchers looked at other cholesterol related numbers from over 27,000 women to see if they were better at predicting future heart problems than a simple total cholesterol number. In most cases women with high LDL cholesterol were high across the board, and the same could be said for those with low values, however a small percentage did not follow the rule. If their LDL cholesterol level was high, one (or more) of the other measures would be below it. Similarly there were women whose LDL cholesterol was low while one or more of the other values measured was high.

Those with low overall cholesterol (LDL-C) but high levels of non-HDL Cholesterol had three times as many cardiovascular events as those with low overall cholesterol and low levels of non-HDL Cholesterol.

Those with high overall cholesterol but low non-HDL-cholesterol had one third as many cardiac events as those whose scores were high for both.

The study showed that cholesterol alone was **not** a good indicator of future heart disease as it over or underestimated the risk for a significant proportion of the population. It also showed that the *size* of LDL particles was related to risk of heart disease with large cholesterol particles to be preferred over small.

In 2017 another study showed that there was no relationship between dietary fat consumption (the food we eat) and the lipid content of our blood.[3]

Confused?

If your doctor says your cholesterol levels are high, you may want to ask for more details to understand why he or she thinks you are at risk. It's clear that cholesterol numbers are not as simple as was once thought, so what can you do to predict your actual risk of heart disease. There are several possible courses of action.

- Do Nothing and wait and see.
- Assume you are at risk and start modifying your behaviour now.
- Assume you are at risk and ask your doctor for medication.
- Ask your doctor for a reliable test that can predict your risk level with accuracy.

Believe it or not, a reliable and accurate test has existed for years, but is only now receiving the attention it deserves.

---

[1] https://www.letsgetchecked.com/articles/what-is-cholesterol-hdl-ldl-and-triglycerides/

[2] https://www.ncbi.nlm.nih.gov/pubmed/24345402

[3] https://www.medicalnewstoday.com/articles/317118.php

6

Which Test Should You Have?

In addition to blood tests there are many ways to screen for heart disease.

These include

- Electrocariograms (ECG)
- Echocardiograms
- Stress testing

Some tests are non-invasive, but others require the insertion of a tube into an artery or something similar, something most of us would want to avoid if possible.

According to Mathew Budoff a professor of medicine at UCLA "the risk calculators we have now are only correct about sixty percent of the time"[1]

One test is changing that. The cardiac calcium score can not only indicate *whether* arteries have plaque deposits, it can measure their extent and make a prediction about the severity of any likely problems. Almost thirty years since it was first developed, the Calcium Score is now part of the American Heart Association's guidelines (from Jan 2019) for cholesterol management. Doctors are now encouraged to use Coronary Artery Calcium scans to look at their patients risk and work out if they need to take any statins.[2]

Calcium scoring grew out of the famous Framington[3] Heart Study. Doctors have used cholesterol levels as a screening method for years. The problem, as Dr Agatston, the inventor of the Calcium score has said is "if you gave statins to everyone, you would be treating a lot of people unnecessarily, but if you only gave it to people with the highest cholesterol you would be missing the majority of people who have heart attacks."[4]

At first the calcium scoring test required expensive super fast CT scanners, but in the years since the test was first developed the availability of the scanners has increased and the cost of the test has gone down to the point where some hospitals and medical centers provide it for $200- $450.

7

What is a Calcium Scoring Test

A CT (computed tomography) scanner produces pictures of your body you can view in almost any cross-section giving doctors an accurate idea of what you look like on the inside without having to cut you open.

The process is not invasive and completely painless. Your doctor will ask you to avoid eating and smoking for about four hours before the test, and you'll have to remove all metal objects, jewelry, dentures, hearings aids, piercings etc. You'll be alone in the room while the scan is performed, but the process will be monitored by a technician and you will be able to speak to them and hear them.

The machine consists of x-ray beams and detectors which rotate around your body and record how much radiation your body has absorbed. The scanner takes pictures and then the table moves. It's very much like splitting your body into thin slices, a computer is required to do the very large number of calculations involved. Modern CT scanners are so fast they can do they whole job in a few seconds.

In a procedure which typically lasts no more than 10 minutes you'll be placed on the table in the right position, propped up by pillows if necessary and some electrodes will be attached to your chest so the technologist can 'see' you're heartbeat. The 'table' of the machine will run through it to verify the path that has been chosen and then, once again to complete the actual scan. As the pictures are taken you'll be asked to hold your breath for around ten to twenty seconds.

A radiologist will then interpret the scan and send a report to your doctor.

If your arteries do have plaque deposits, there will be calcium in the older deposits and this is what shows up on the scan. Tests have shown that this is the single most accurate way to predict heart attacks even when patients have absolutely no symptoms. The relationship between this calcium score and heart disease has been established in several studies.[1]

As a result the calcium score is now recom-

The Heart Test That Could Save Your Life

mended by most doctors for those patients at medium risk or where statins have been prescribed and the patient is, for one reason or another, reluctant to take them.

Is there a downside?

Of course. There always is.

1. Many insurance companies do not cover the cost of the test (although this is changing and the test itself is not usually too expensive)

2. The test involves a low dose of radiation which makes it inappropriate for certain patients (pregnant women, for example) however as the amount of radiation involved is roughly equivalent to that of a mammogram, most doctors consider it harmless.

8

Who Uses the Calcium Score?

One area in which the calcium score has already made an impact is space travel.

With limited medicines, medical equipment and expertise, astronauts in space are interdependent. A major medical problem affecting one individual can compromise the entire mission leading to mission failure and the possibility of multiple fatalities. For this reasons NASA does a great deal of research into the effects of long term space travel which have been found similar to those of aging.

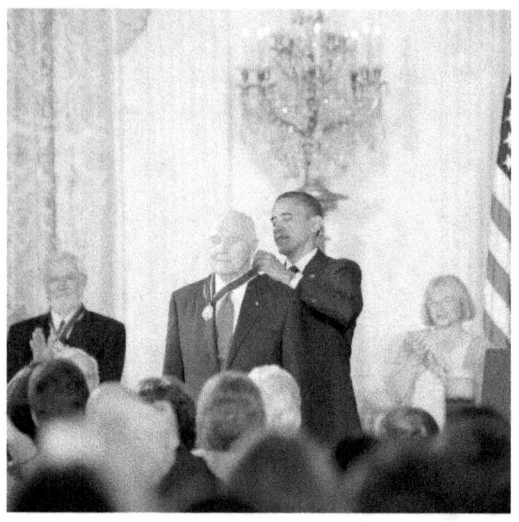

John Glenn, one of the USA's original group of astronauts and the fifth man in space, receiving the Presidential Medal of Freedom from President Obama

Ever since the first astronauts were recruited, their overall health has been a major issue and health screening is still a major part of admission to the astronaut corps. A recent suggestion has been that only those with a calcium score of 0 should be accepted.

Many risk factors for coronary artery disease increase naturally with age and this could bias conventional selection procedures in favor of the young, ruling out the use of more experienced staff, a factor NASA considers could be crucial to the success of any space mission. Use of the calcium score will hopefully prevent heart-healthy trained astronauts from being denied flight status and pave the way for their inclusion on crucial long term spaceflights such as mission to Mars.

Unsurprisingly NASA is not alone. Airline pilots, like astronauts, carry the burden of other people's lives. For this reason their health is checked regularly and many airlines do not allow pilots over a certain age to fly which, once again, excludes the most experienced pilots from flight status.

The International Civil Aviation Authority (ICAO) sets the retirement age for pilots at 65, while many airlines set the age at sixty. This causes problems for pilots who find themselves out of a job before being old enough to qualify for a pension.

Due largely to the considerable shortage of pilots, some aviation authorities (Japan, for example) have increased that age to 67. At present calcium scores are not used to determine whether a pilot passes the required medical but the matter is in discussion and for good reason. Experienced pilots are more likely to have knowledge of flying which is not dependent on the automated systems younger pilots trained with. Furthermore, a recent study showed that the performance of experienced pilots declined less over time than the performance of those in a lower age group. As a result expect to see the calcium score feature in many of these crucial operational medical exams where it will, hopefully, allow experience to be retained.

A great deal of information about aging in space was gathered from experiments run by John Glenn, one of the very first astronauts and the fifth man in space. In 1998 John Glenn, then aged 77, returned to space as a payload specialist on STS-95 to participate in studies of the aging process which has many similarities with long term spaceflight. Perhaps NASA's adoption of the calcium score as part of their screening tests will allow more experienced astronauts to return to space over the coming decades.

Note: John Glenn died in December 2016 aged 95. He retained his pilot's license until aged 90.

9

Why Don't We Take Steps to Help Ourselves?

Given the prevalence of heart disease, you might wonder why we don't all take as many precautions as we can. Why don't we live 'heart-friendly' lives, for example?

The truth is it's difficult to work out what a heart-friendly life would be like. Any google search will tell you about 'heart friendly diets' 'heart friendly foods' and the internet is full of advice on how to stay healthy. Given that every year around 735,000 Americans have a heart attack there's only one possible conclusion. Either healthy heart-friendly living doesn't work, or we're just ignoring the information. For just over a quarter of a million people a year, their first heart attack is also their last. They may have meant to exercise or mind their diet, but since cardiovascular disease has very few symptoms in the early stages, we all feel the same way.

- It won't happen to me.
- I'll deal with it if and when I get symptoms.

For many people the first symptom of heart disease is a heart attack and all that entails.

There is pain and inconvenience as a minimum. You may be left incapable of doing some things you did before. You might even die. What about the people you'll leave behind?

You owe it to them, the people you love and the people who love you, to pay attention. To learn about the risks and most of all, to take action.

10

Why Do We Ignore Medical Advice

The internet is full of medical advice. Who has the time to stay up to date? What's more, the advice that reaches the media is often quite different to the actual results of a clinical trial. Medical jargon creates a barrier between doctor and patient, researcher and reporter. Not many of us can read the research papers as written and understand both what is said *and* its implications. Reporters, sadly, are as guilty as the rest of us. Confronted with the results of some medical research they simplify, sometimes to the point where accuracy is compromised.

Medicine is a complex subject. What you hear in the media, the newspapers and blogs, is often far from accurate. This leads to another reason to ignore medical advice.

Lack of Trust

Type any medical query into the internet and you'll find a lot of the response is in the form of ads. There's so much money to be made by selling drugs and treatment

it's not surprising we don't trust what we're told. The market for statins (a common treatment for cardiovascular disease) is worth $1 trillion alone. Just think about those zeros for a moment, all twelve of them. One trillion is so much money it's almost impossible to spend! You'd have to spend one million dollars a *day* every day since the foundation of the Roman Empire! Many medical studies are funded by the food or pharmaceutical companies who stand to make this kind of money from their products. You may have to think about their claims carefully to understand what you are dealing with.

For example - a food described as 'heart healthy' may not actually lead to a healthier heart, it may just be less *unhealthy* than the previous version. A lot depends on regulation which in turn can depend on influence.

The claim 'heart healthy' is biased to the food manufacturers advantage, and the same can be true of drugs and procedures. Doctors gain information on the drugs they prescribe from drug company employees whose job is to sell. Most doctors believe that their medical advice is entirely independent of any pharmaceutical company's influence, but when that influence extends to the specification of recommended guidelines the doctor should follow, it takes courage to go against the norm. In today's world the information doctors receive from drug companies could well be biased.

One of the biggest obstacles, when dealing with medical problems, is access to accurate unbiased information and advice.

Contradiction:

If you're over forty you've almost certainly seen medical advice contradict itself. And when you think about it this is reasonable. Medical research advances year by year and some ideas which appeared correct will inevitably be found to be wrong. Who is to say it won't happen again?

Cholesterol is a good example. For years heart patients were told to avoid eating eggs because of the high cholesterol content of their yokes. Today doctors say there is no danger in one egg a day but they can't recommend more.

The reason's simple. Subsequent studies have shown there is no relationship between cholesterol consumed in food and the cholesterol in your blood. Why then do doctors appear to tell us not to eat more than one a day? Simply because they have no evidence one way or another, but rather than say 'you're on your own' because they don't actually know, they recommend one egg a day and we assume the rest. One study says yes, the next study says no. Even within the medical profession standards vary.

Who should you believe?

Negativity

Medical advice always seems to be framed in negative terms. It's all about what you give up, rarely about what you gain, it's as though the advice has been written for us to ignore.

Look at the advice doctors give to the over fifties. Exercise, they say, as though it's easy to change the habits of a lifetime. Join a gym, get a personal trainer. Leaving aside the simple problems, like the expense and finding the time, they seem vague on the reasons we should do so. Somewhere the message gets lost.

You may have elderly relatives with physical

limitations like walking, bending, even brushing their hair, most people do. We all begin to lose muscle mass in our forties and doctors say we can slow down the degradation by doing strength training exercises, yet a recent report from the CDC shows that only 23% of Americans try to meet the CDC guidelines of 150 minutes of exercise a week.

Why is that?

It could be because change is hard. A new exercise regime means acquiring new habits and that is not an easy thing to do, but if you were told that lifting weights could *reverse* the infirmity of age, give you back your strength, wouldn't you feel more motivated to try? You really do regain muscle mass and strength when you exercise, which is far better than simply losing it more slowly.

11

What are the Treatments for Heart Disease?

There are many possible treatments for cardiovascular disease. Your doctor will suggest the appropriate course of action based on your risk of future heart attacks.

These include

- Lifestyle changes - exercise and Diet
- Maintaining a healthy weight
- Drugs - like statins
- Surgery to bypass the heart
- Surgery to open the blocked artery.

12

Which Diet Should You Follow?

Although doctors may disagree on the detail of which foods are best for your heart they are agreed that diet can make a big difference.

Your heart is a muscle, like your biceps and triceps. A diet to improve your general health and fitness will also help your heart. Foods high in antioxidants are part of every heart health diet plan, but other foods are more controversial, no more so than fat.

Some diets insist that fats are good for you and olive oils, we're told, is almost miraculous. For most of these sugar in all its forms, including fruit, is the food type to avoid.

Other diets praise olive oil but insist in the use of low fat dairy products, for example, while allowing the consumption of plant based fats like avocado and nuts.

Yet others insist that olive oil and avocados are to be avoided at all cost, and the removal of all fats from any diet is not at all easy, not least because many vitamins A, D, E and K are all fat soluble. Without consuming fat we simply won't get enough of them.

13

Different Approaches to Diet

Most doctor's recommend a Mediterranean style diet with an emphasis on salad and olive oil dressings, fish at least twice a week and fruit and vegetables daily. Where recommendations differ is when it comes to carbohydrate rich foods like bread, rice and pasta, fats like butter and milk and of course, eggs.

The DASH Diet.

Similar to the Mediterranean diet the DASH diet emphasises the use of fruits and vegetables and provides a simple rule: look at the color the deepest colors are the healthiest.

High on the list are:

- Strawberries and blueberries. Three servings a week are said to make a dramatic reduction to heart attack risk.
- Dark Greens, like spinach and kale. Since these are among the 'dirty dozen'[1] be sure to clean them properly or go for genuinely organic.

For full details of the DASH diet, visit the National Heart Lung and Blood Institute[2]

While the DASH Diet is highly regarded, researchers agree it isn't easy to stick to and tests have shown it to be less effective than other diet plans. As a result you might want to choose a different approach.

Low Carbohydrate Diets

High levels of cholesterol and triglycerides are associated with blocked arteries and inflammation. A 1984 study showed a relationship between lowering cholesterol and reducing the number of heart attacks. The best thing about it was that no drugs were needed, just a change of diet. The American Heart Association recommended a low-fat high-carbohydrate diet to alter cholesterol levels, and in many cases this did produce a small improvement, however as Dr Agatston (who created the calcium score AND the South Beach diet) puts it

'there were no convincing studies showing that the American Heart Association diet saved lives.'[3]

Low Carbohydrate diets were also intended to battle heart disease, lower blood pressure, cholesterol and weight, and introduced the idea of **insulin resistance**. When your blood sugar rises, as it does when you eat carbohydrates, your pancreas detects the rise and releases insulin to 'mop up' the sugar. If the amount of insulin released is high, the result is a sudden drop in your blood sugar level, setting off your body's alert system where, despite what you have already eaten, you want more. As a result, you overeat and get fat.

This idea was revolutionary in its claim that carbohydrates, rather than fats, were the bogeyman of foods and made the solution seem simple; cut the number of carbohydrates you eat, and don't let your insulin or blood sugar spike.

These diets are typically divided into stages, with the first, extremely restrictive stage banning all carbohydrates, including bread, while allowing eggs and bacon. A 2015 study of the Atkins diet[4] found that those on low carb diets experienced greater weight loss that those on low fat diets but also had an increase in LDL *and* HDL cholesterol. Some doctors reject the use of low carb diets on that basis, however more recent research suggests that it isn't the absolute level of LDL or HDL cholesterol that matters, but the relationship between the two.

One diet which builds on the low carb regime of the Atkins diet is the South Beach diet, which like Atkins, was devised by a cardiologist (Dr Agatston) whose patients found the Dash diet didn't work for them. The South Beach Diet depends on the idea of Glycemic Index and Glycemic Load.

Glycemic Index and Glycemic Load Based Diets

The *glycemic index* (GI) of a food is a measure of how fast 25 or 50 grams of carbohydrate will increase your blood sugar level. For example, the glycemic index of carrots in 131. However this measurement does not take into account the *amount* of carbohydrate in a food and so the concept of *Glycemic Load* (GL) was born. For example, there are only 8g of carbohydrate in a serving of carrots. You can calculate the GL for that portion of carrots using the GI (47) time the amount of carbohydrate (8) and expressing the result as a percentage

Glycemic Load = 47 x 8 / 100 = 3.76

This number can be used to compare foods and is useful in modifying and adapting low carb diet plans to your individual requirements. Using values like GL it is possible to divide carbohydrates into different 'camps'. Many criticised the Atkins diet's rejection of fruit, for example, because of fruit's high carbohydrate content. However, this is mostly stored as fructose which releases sugar into the body far more slowly than glucose and this is easy to see if you do the calculation.

Compare, for example, watermelon, which has a high glycemic index (72) and, as a fruit, is not permitted on the Atkins diet. The carbohydrate content of a portion is only 5g, with the result that the GL is less that 4.

Rice has a far lower glycemic index (64) but a much higher carbohydrate content (25g in a 100g portion) giving a GL of 16.

To find the glycemic index and glycemic load of many foods you can simply search the internet but there are a large number of diet apps (such as Carb Manager) you can use on your smartphone to provide all the information you need.

All doctors agree that weight loss reduces the risk of heart disease. If one diet plan doesn't suit you, there are many more to try!

14

Specific Food Types

What is an Antioxidant

Antioxidants help to slow down or prevent cell damage known as oxidative stress.

There are two types. Some antioxidants are chemicals added to food and other products to prevent their decay. The second type of antioxidant occurs naturally in food and in the body. Vitamins C and E are B examples of this type as is the mineral selenium. Other antioxidants include carotenoids lycopene, zeaxanthin, lutein and beta-carotene. Almost all plants contain antioxidants, you can also find antioxidant vitamins in eggs, legumes and nuts.

Reactive Oxygen Species (free radicals)

These are unstable molecules which contain oxygen and react with other molecules very easily. If reactive oxygen species are allowed to build up in cells they can damage DNA, RNA, proteins and may cause cell death.

Oxidative Stress

Occurs when your body's production of reactivate oxygen species exceeds its ability to clean them up. (Detoxify them)

Olive Oil

Doctors are agreed, olive oil 'improves cardio-vascular risk'. Olive oil is perfect in salad dressings, or as a dip for bread. Choose extra virgin olive oil as this has not been refined, but be careful many oils in the United States are labelled extra virgin when they're not. To be sure, check the brand you want to buy against the latest consumer reports. In 2015, brands like Coalvita, Lucini and California Olive Ranch were found to be genuinely extra virgin. Olive oil does not have a high 'smoke point' which means it should only be used at low temperatures or most of the good things in it degrade.

· · ·

Avocado Oil has a higher smoke point than Olive Oil and is hence better for cooking, but the downside is expense.

Peanut Oil has one of the high smoke points as does Sesame oil. Both can be used for high heat cooking.

Walnut Oil and Flaxseed oil both have low smoke points and work week as dressings.

Avocados

Contain monounsaturated fatty acids just like olive oil. They also contain phytochemicals which work as antioxidants. Best of all, avocados taste good with a simple oil dressing and take next to no time to prepare.

Other similar heart healthy foods are garlic, onions, asparagus, brussels sprouts, cabbage, cauliflower, kale, parsley and watercress.

Spices can also be useful as heart therapy, for example cinnamon, cardamom and curcumin are all heart healthy.

Vitamin E

In most cases your body absorbs more of any vitamin from food than it would from a supplement. Vitamins typically require other vitamins and minerals to support their absorption. While the right quantities can usually be found in food, this is not the case when you take a single supplement.

This is why doctors and nutritionists emphasize healthy eating over taking supplements. In most cases your body absorbs more of any vitamin from food than it would from a supplement. Vitamins typically require other vitamins and minerals to support their absorption. While the right quantities can usually be found in food, this is not the case when you take a single supplement. This is why doctors and nutritionists emphasize healthy eating over taking supplements.

However, in the case of some vitamins, it's not easy to get a high dose from food. Vitamin E is an example. Doctors feel levels of up to 800 IU per day are known to be safe and various trials have shown vitamin E to be able to reduce the risk of heart disease, but most fruits and vegetables store vitamin E in small quantities[1] making it difficult to obtain a therapeutic dose from diet alone. In this case a supplement might be considered.

CoEnzyme Q10 is a vitamin like substance thought to reduce blood pressure. There is some suggestion that Coenzyme Q10 is depleted in those people who take statins. If you are on statin medication you may require a supplement.

Omega 3 Oils are popular supplements and many believe these can improve heart health, however most doctors agree that it is far better to get your Omega 3 from food sources than from supplements. Sources of omega 3 include

- Oily fish (like salmon or mackerel)
- Nuts and seeds (e.g. walnuts)
- Oils such as flaxseed oil and canola oil
- Some fortified foods like eggs and yogurt

Avocados also contain Omega 3 oils but to a much lesser extent.

Always tell your doctor about any supplements you take as these may interfere with your medication. For example heart patients prescribed warfarin to reduce blood clotting may find coenzyme Q10 decreases its effectiveness.

15

Drug Treatment

The most common drug treatment for heart disease is a type of drug called a **statin**. These were discovered due to the work on cholesterol done by Dr's Brown and Goldstein.

Statins are enormously popular drugs, however they are also controversial. While millions take them every day without problems, there have been claims of unpleasant side effects from taking them and though many studies have said these problems are not significant, the studies themselves are controversial.

Lipitor is the brand name of a popular statin called atorvastatin which was patented in 1986 and approved ten years later. By 2006, Lipitor had made $13 billion dollars in the USA alone. By 2016 it was the third most prescribed medication in the USA and has retained that position[1]. Over 35 million people in the USA take statins every day, and 8 million people in the UK. These drugs are popular all over the world but the various statins have been controversial since their introduction and there has recently been a call for a complete and transparent enquiry into their use[2] in the UK. Some patients complain of severe side effects, such as muscle pain and cramps or even liver disease. Others inside the medical profession claim that statins do little good and asa result represent money which could be better spent elsewhere. According to Dr Aseem Malhotra,

---

"If you strip down the statin trials to their moving parts, the data actually reveals that, even in those who have established heart disease, the benefits are very small. Even in this high risk group, the average increase in life expectancy from taking the drug religiously for five years is a meagre four days[3]"

Dr Aseem Malhotra

At the center of the controversy is the issue of transparency. The data from clinical trials of these drugs has not been made available by the pharmaceutical companies making it impossible to judge whether they are as effective as claimed.

If your doctor prescribes statins and you suffer side effects, make sure to tell your doctor and don't simply stop taking them. There are alternatives, but your doctor can't solve your problem if he or she doesn't know.

16

One Hundred and Fifty Minutes of Fun

Exercise is another important component of a heart healthy life. Guidelines indicate you need 150 minutes of exercise a week to see a benefit from it.

In a recent Korean[1] study of patients with and without heart disease results showed exercise was *more* beneficial to those *with* heart disease than to those without. There was a 14% reduction in the risk of death over the six years of the study.

Heart Healthy Exercises Should Cover:

- Aerobic exercise. This gives your heart a good workout and makes perfect sense given that your heart is a muscle like any

other. A brisk walk, swimming, jogging or cycling are all a good idea. The recommendation is for 150 minutes of this type of exercise each week.
- Strength Training builds back muscle mass you have lost. It also lowers blood sugar and improves posture and balance, so buy some weights and learn to use them. The ideal weight is one you can lift without effort around six or seven times. To build you muscles
- Stretching Exercises help your muscle stay flexible and reduce pain from stiffness and cramp.
- Balance Exercises help to prevent falls and will also give you more confidence. You'll do a lot of balance training if you take up Yoga or Tai Chi.

While 150 minutes may sound like a lot you can spread it over a week and do 20 minutes or so per day, or divide it among the working days and exercise for 30 minutes 5 days a week.

Afterword

There was a time, quite long ago, when patients blindly followed their doctors recommendations.

Now so many treatments involve self help, it's impossible to take that attitude. Without understanding what your doctor tells you, you can't make all the necessary lifestyle changes.

I can't imagine how a doctor feels when they hear a patient say 'I read on the internet' but the old days are gone. Decisions about your health should be your decisions, not your doctor's, his job is to provide advice so your decision can be properly informed or at the very least so you can give informed consent to his proposed treatment plan.

When you see a doctor, take someone with you. Write a list of questions you want to ask, write down the answers and don't feel it's wrong.

Afterword

Everyone leaves their doctors office feeling slightly numb, no matter how much money they have or how much education. Doctors need many skills and some, though very skilled in medicine, are just not good at talking to people. If that's the case with your doctor help them out or get a new doctor.

Heart disease is a real threat, but you **can** take action. You can change your diet, reduce your weight, take more exercise. You may have no symptoms of heart disease, but most people don't. Why not be safe rather than sorry and just assume you are at risk?

If your doctor has already suggested medication ask 'Why?' and work to understand the answer. If you can't find it in you to stick to the diet or take some medication you know you need, get yourself tested. Ask for a Calcium Score. Find out your actual risk and then own it. Make time. Put in the effort.

Don't make your family wish you had.

Yours

L M Clay (hearttest@yahoo.com)

Medical Terms You Should Understand

Arteriosclerosis is stiffness of the large arteries surrounding the heart and is a common side-effect of aging. Scientists have also discovered a genetic component which makes someone more likely to suffer from the this form of cardiovascular disease.[1]

CVD is cardiovascular disease

Hypercholesteremia - High cholesterol levels

Lipoprotein - any soluble protein which combines with or transports fat in the blood.

LDL Low Density Lipoprotein - often known as 'bad' cholesterol This number is frequently regarded as the primary indicator of elevated risk of heart disease. Also known as LDL-C

LDL Particle Number (LDL-P) the number of LDL particles in the blood.

HDL High Density Lipoprotein - often known as 'good' cholesterol is responsible for transporting cholesterol to the liver and hence out of the body.

Plaque A fatty substance which can build up on the inside of your arterial walls causing atherosclerosis.

Statins - the drug most often prescribed for Cardiovascular disease. It was designed to control cholesterol levels. Lipitor is one example.

Atherosclerosis: The build up of plaque on the inside of artery walls.

Echocardiogram - a test which uses sound waves to look at your heart muscle.

Notes

Introduction

1. https://www.cdc.gov/heartdisease/facts.htm

2. What is a Heart Attack?

1. https://www.health.harvard.edu/a_to_z/heart-attack-myocardial-infarction-a-to-z
2. Blood is more valuable than gold, weight for weight, but sadly does not last nearly as long.
3. Fun Fact - this makes them completely different from red blood cells in birds and fish where the cell does have a nucleus.

3. Why Do Arteries Become Blocked?

1. https://www.health.com/cholesterol/dr-raj-cholesterol-questions
2. https://www.webmd.com/heart-disease/clogged-arteries-arterial-plaque#3

4. Does Everyone Get Heart Disease?

1. https://www.crossfit.com/essentials/impact-of-the-diet-heart-hypothesis
2. Cohen E, et al. Americans have been following dietary

guidelines, coincident with the rise in obesity. *Nutrition.* 31.5(2015): 727-732.

6. Which Test Should You Have?

1. https://www.dicardiology.com/article/ct-calcium-scoring-becoming-key-risk-factor-assessment
2. https://www.dicardiology.com/content/blogs/how-agatston-calcium-score-was-created-and-its-impact-heart-attack-prevention
3. https://www.framinghamheartstudy.org/fhs-risk-functions/hard-coronary-heart-disease-10-year-risk/
4. https://www.dicardiology.com/content/blogs/how-agatston-calcium-score-was-created-and-its-impact-heart-attack-prevention

7. What is a Calcium Scoring Test

1. https://www.sciencedirect.com/science/article/pii/-S1936878X19306175

13. Different Approaches to Diet

1. Foods most likely to be pesticide laden.
2. https://www.nhlbi.nih.gov/health-topics/dash-eating-plan
3. Agatston, The South Beach Diet, p9
4. One of the first low carbohydrate diet plans

14. Specific Food Types

1. An apple, for example, has 0.3 mg

15. Drug Treatment

1. https://clincalc.com/DrugStats/Top300Drugs.aspx
2. https://www.europeanscientist.com/en/features/do-statins-really-work-who-benefits-who-has-the-power-to-cover-up-the-side-effects/
3. https://bmjopen.bmj.com/content/6/3/e010500

16. One Hundred and Fifty Minutes of Fun

1. https://academic.oup.com/eurheartj/advance-article/doi/10.1093/eurheartj/ehz564/5552546

Medical Terms You Should Understand

1. https://www.ahajournals.org/doi/abs/10.1161/ATVBAHA.119.312405

www.ingramcontent.com/pod-product-compliance
Lightning Source LLC
Chambersburg PA
CBHW070451220526
45466CB00004B/1798